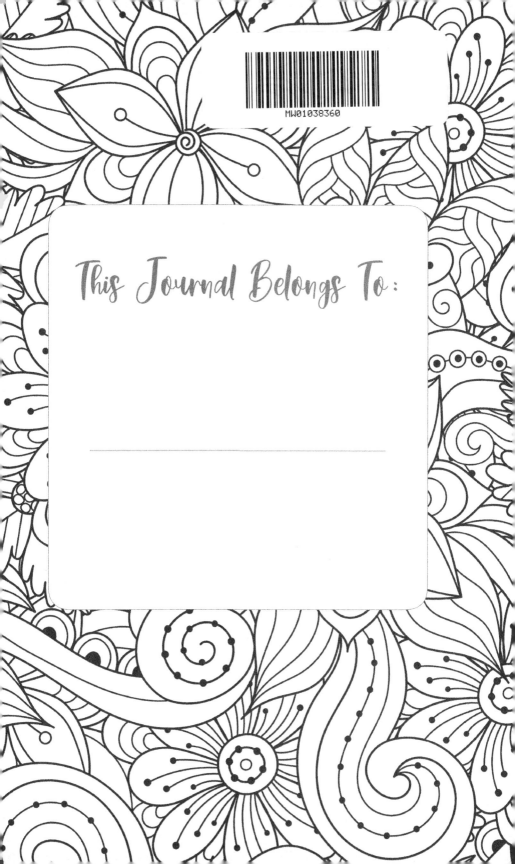

MW01038360

This Journal Belongs To:

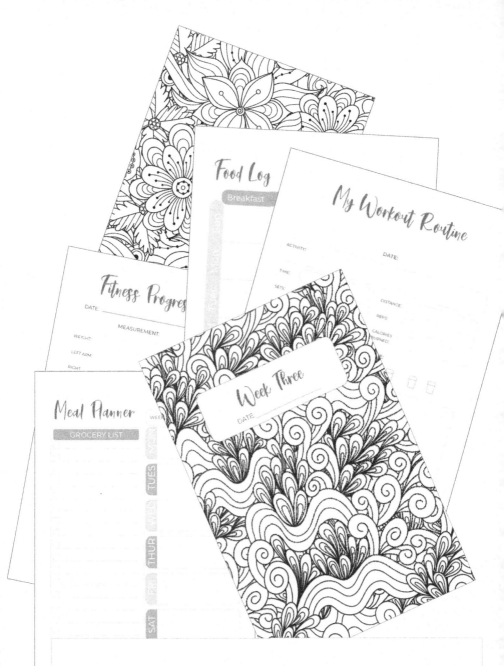

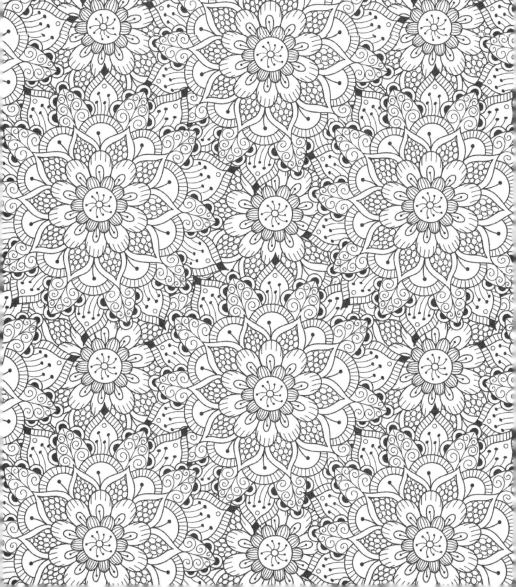

Week One

DATE: _____

This Week's Goals

FITNESS TO DO   M   T   W   T   F   S   S

Fitness Progress Tracker

STARTING MEASUREMENTS

DATE: _____

WEIGHT +/-

LEFT BICEP

RIGHT BICEP

CHEST

WAIST

HIPS

LEFT THIGH

RIGHT THIGH

LEFT CALF

RIGHT CALF

My Workout Routine

DATE:

ACTIVITY:

TIME:

DISTANCE:

SETS:

REPS:

WEIGHT USED:

CALORIES BURNED:

WATER INTAKE:

NOTES:

Just Breathe

My Workout Routine

DATE:

ACTIVITY:

TIME:

DISTANCE:

SETS:

REPS:

WEIGHT USED:

CALORIES BURNED:

WATER INTAKE:

NOTES:

Just Breathe

My Workout Routine

DATE:

ACTIVITY:

TIME:

DISTANCE:

SETS:

REPS:

WEIGHT USED:

CALORIES BURNED:

WATER INTAKE:

NOTES:

Just Breathe

My Workout Routine

DATE:

ACTIVITY:

TIME:

DISTANCE:

SETS:

REPS:

WEIGHT USED:

CALORIES BURNED:

WATER INTAKE:

NOTES:

Just Breathe

Meal Planner

WEEK OF

GROCERY LIST

- [ ]
- [ ]
- [ ]
- [ ]
- [ ]
- [ ]
- [ ]
- [ ]
- [ ]
- [ ]
- [ ]
- [ ]
- [ ]
- [ ]
- [ ]
- [ ]
- [ ]
- [ ]

MON

TUES

WED

THUR

FRI

SAT

SUN

Food Log

WEEK OF

	Breakfast	Lunch	Dinner	Snacks
Sun				
Mon				
Tues				
Wed				
Thur				
Fri				
Sat				

Thoughts...

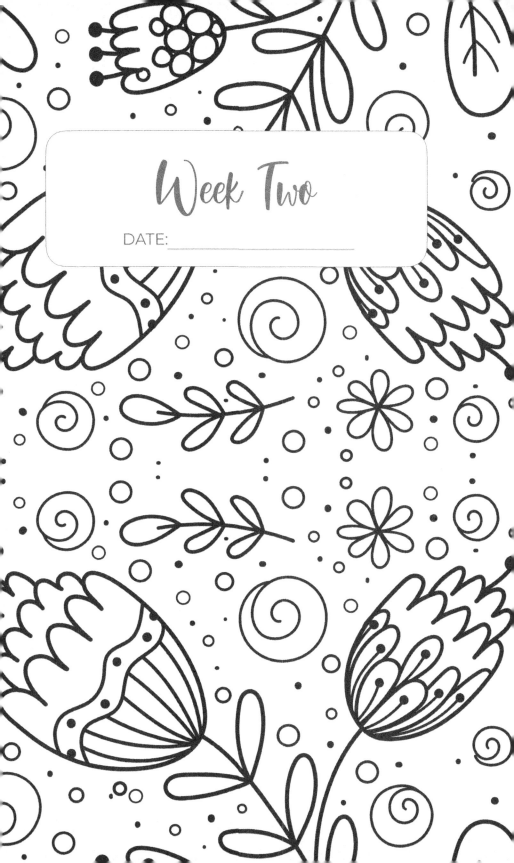

Week Two

DATE: _____

This Week's Goals

FITNESS TO DO   **M**   **T**   **W**   **T**   **F**   **S**   **S**

Fitness Progress Tracker

DATE: ....

	MEASUREMENT:	LOSS/GAIN:
WEIGHT:		
LEFT ARM:		
RIGHT ARM:		
CHEST:		
WAIST:		
HIPS:		
LEFT THIGH:		
RIGHT THIGH:		

How's It Going?

Good things TAKES TIME

My Workout Routine

DATE:

ACTIVITY:

TIME:

DISTANCE:

SETS:

REPS:

WEIGHT USED:

CALORIES BURNED:

WATER INTAKE:

NOTES:

Just Breathe

My Workout Routine

DATE:

ACTIVITY:

TIME:

DISTANCE:

SETS:

REPS:

WEIGHT USED:

CALORIES BURNED:

WATER INTAKE:

NOTES:

Just Breathe

My Workout Routine

DATE:

ACTIVITY:

TIME:

DISTANCE:

SETS:

REPS:

WEIGHT USED:

CALORIES BURNED:

WATER INTAKE:

NOTES:

Just Breathe

My Workout Routine

DATE:

ACTIVITY:

TIME:

DISTANCE:

SETS:

REPS:

WEIGHT USED:

CALORIES BURNED:

WATER INTAKE:

NOTES:

Just Breathe

Meal Planner

WEEK OF

GROCERY LIST

- [ ] _____
- [ ] _____
- [ ] _____
- [ ] _____
- [ ] _____
- [ ] _____
- [ ] _____
- [ ] _____
- [ ] _____
- [ ] _____
- [ ] _____
- [ ] _____
- [ ] _____
- [ ] _____
- [ ] _____
- [ ] _____
- [ ] _____
- [ ] _____

MON

TUES

WED

THUR

FRI

SAT

SUN

Food Log

WEEK OF

	Breakfast	Lunch	Dinner	Snacks
Sun				
Mon				
Tues				
Wed				
Thur				
Fri				
Sat				

Thoughts. . .

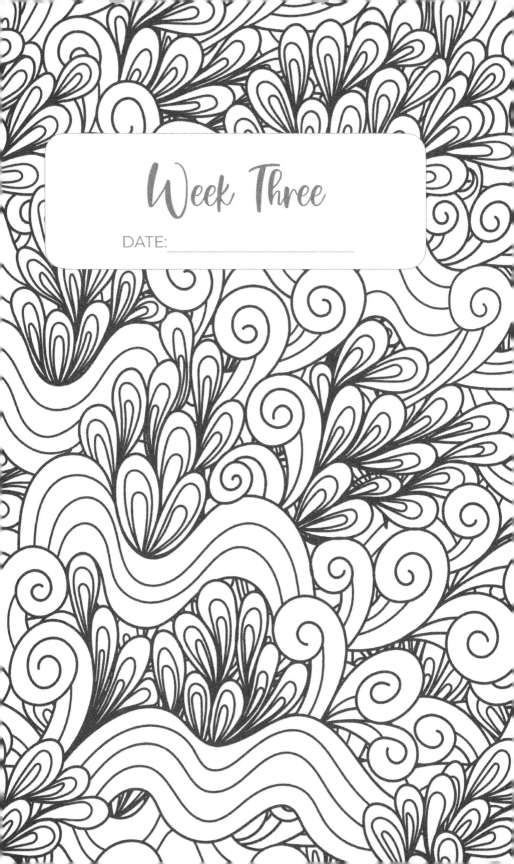

Week Three

DATE: _____

This Week's Goals

FITNESS TO DO   **M   T   W   T   F   S   S**

Fitness Progress Tracker

DATE: _____

	MEASUREMENT:	LOSS/GAIN:
WEIGHT:		
LEFT ARM:		
RIGHT ARM:		
CHEST:		
WAIST:		
HIPS:		
LEFT THIGH:		
RIGHT THIGH:		

How's It Going?

Good things TAKE TIME

My Workout Routine

DATE:

ACTIVITY:

TIME:

DISTANCE:

SETS:

REPS:

WEIGHT USED:

CALORIES BURNED:

WATER INTAKE:

NOTES:

Just Breathe

My Workout Routine

DATE:

ACTIVITY:

TIME:

DISTANCE:

SETS:

REPS:

WEIGHT USED:

CALORIES BURNED:

WATER INTAKE:

NOTES:

Just Breathe

My Workout Routine

DATE:

ACTIVITY:

TIME:

DISTANCE:

SETS:

REPS:

WEIGHT USED:

CALORIES BURNED:

WATER INTAKE:

NOTES:

Just Breathe

My Workout Routine

DATE:

ACTIVITY:

TIME:

DISTANCE:

SETS:

REPS:

WEIGHT
USED:

CALORIES
BURNED:

WATER INTAKE:

NOTES:

Just
Breathe

Meal Planner

WEEK OF

GROCERY LIST

- [ ]
- [ ]
- [ ]
- [ ]
- [ ]
- [ ]
- [ ]
- [ ]
- [ ]
- [ ]
- [ ]
- [ ]
- [ ]
- [ ]
- [ ]
- [ ]
- [ ]
- [ ]
- [ ]
- [ ]

MON

TUES

WED

THUR

FRI

SAT

SUN

Food Log

WEEK OF

	Breakfast	Lunch	Dinner	Snacks
Sun				
Mon				
Tues				
Wed				
Thur				
Fri				
Sat				

Thoughts . . .

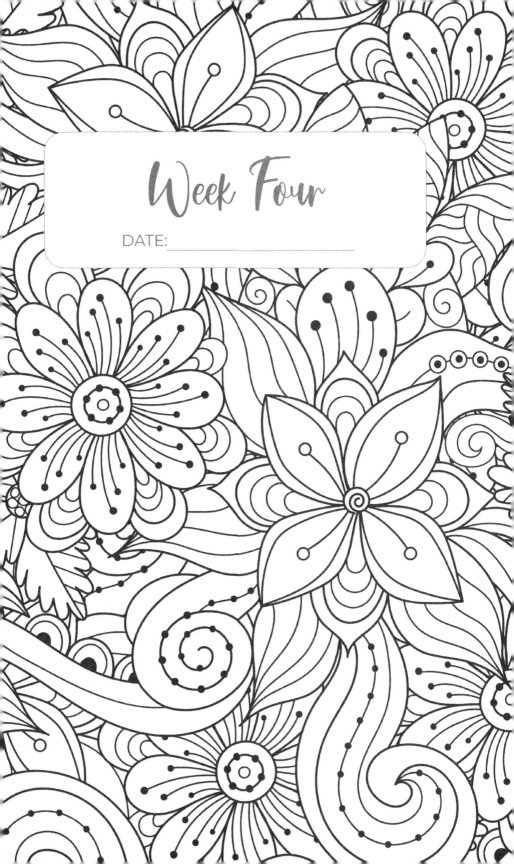

Week Four

DATE: _____

This Week's Goals

FITNESS TO DO	M	T	W	T	F	S	S

Fitness Progress Tracker

DATE: _____

	MEASUREMENT:	LOSS/GAIN:
WEIGHT:		
LEFT ARM:		
RIGHT ARM:		
CHEST:		
WAIST:		
HIPS:		
LEFT THIGH:		
RIGHT THIGH:		

How's It Going?

Good things TAKE TIME

My Workout Routine

DATE:

ACTIVITY:

TIME:

DISTANCE:

SETS:

REPS:

WEIGHT USED:

CALORIES BURNED:

WATER INTAKE:

NOTES:

Just Breathe

My Workout Routine

DATE:

ACTIVITY:

TIME:

DISTANCE:

SETS:

REPS:

WEIGHT USED:

CALORIES BURNED:

WATER INTAKE:

NOTES:

Just Breathe

My Workout Routine

DATE:

ACTIVITY:

TIME:

DISTANCE:

SETS:

REPS:

WEIGHT USED:

CALORIES BURNED:

WATER INTAKE:

NOTES:

Just Breathe

My Workout Routine

DATE:

ACTIVITY:

TIME:

DISTANCE:

SETS:

REPS:

WEIGHT USED:

CALORIES BURNED:

WATER INTAKE:

NOTES:

Just Breathe

Meal Planner

WEEK OF

GROCERY LIST

- [ ]
- [ ]
- [ ]
- [ ]
- [ ]
- [ ]
- [ ]
- [ ]
- [ ]
- [ ]
- [ ]
- [ ]
- [ ]
- [ ]
- [ ]
- [ ]
- [ ]
- [ ]
- [ ]
- [ ]
- [ ]

MON

TUES

WED

THUR

FRI

SAT

SUN

Food Log

WEEK OF

	Breakfast	Lunch	Dinner	Snacks
Sun				
Mon				
Tues				
Wed				
Thur				
Fri				
Sat				

Thoughts. . .

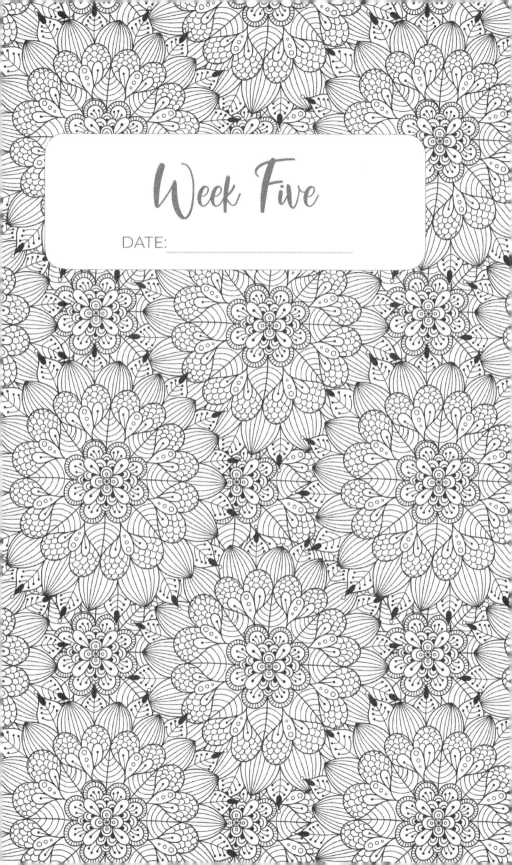

Week Five

DATE:_____

This Week's Goals

FITNESS TO DO   M   T   W   T   F   S   S

Fitness Progress Tracker

DATE: _____

	MEASUREMENT:	LOSS/GAIN:
WEIGHT:		
LEFT ARM:		
RIGHT ARM:		
CHEST:		
WAIST:		
HIPS:		
LEFT THIGH:		
RIGHT THIGH:		

How's It Going?

Good things TAKE TIME

My Workout Routine

DATE:

ACTIVITY:

TIME:

DISTANCE:

SETS:

REPS:

WEIGHT USED:

CALORIES BURNED:

WATER INTAKE:

NOTES:

Just
Breathe

My Workout Routine

DATE:

ACTIVITY:

TIME:

DISTANCE:

SETS:

REPS:

WEIGHT USED:

CALORIES BURNED:

WATER INTAKE:

NOTES:

Just Breathe

My Workout Routine

DATE:

ACTIVITY:

TIME:

DISTANCE:

SETS:

REPS:

WEIGHT USED:

CALORIES BURNED:

WATER INTAKE:

NOTES:

Just Breathe

My Workout Routine

DATE:

ACTIVITY:

TIME:

DISTANCE:

SETS:

REPS:

WEIGHT USED:

CALORIES BURNED:

WATER INTAKE:

NOTES:

Just Breathe

Meal Planner

WEEK OF

GROCERY LIST

- [ ]
- [ ]
- [ ]
- [ ]
- [ ]
- [ ]
- [ ]
- [ ]
- [ ]
- [ ]
- [ ]
- [ ]
- [ ]
- [ ]
- [ ]
- [ ]
- [ ]
- [ ]
- [ ]

MON

TUES

WED

THUR

FRI

SAT

SUN

Food Log

WEEK OF

	Breakfast	Lunch	Dinner	Snacks
Sun				
Mon				
Tues				
Wed				
Thur				
Fri				
Sat				

Thoughts. . .

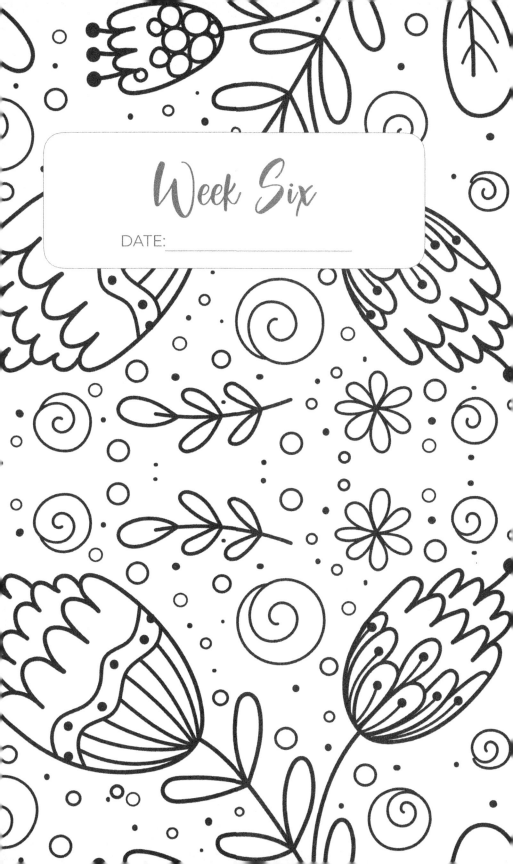

Week Six

DATE: _____

This Week's Goals

FITNESS TO DO   M   T   W   T   F   S   S

Fitness Progress Tracker

DATE: _____

	MEASUREMENT:	LOSS/GAIN:
WEIGHT:		
LEFT ARM:		
RIGHT ARM:		
CHEST:		
WAIST:		
HIPS:		
LEFT THIGH:		
RIGHT THIGH:		

How's It Going?

Good things TAKE TIME

My Workout Routine

DATE:

ACTIVITY:

TIME:

DISTANCE:

SETS:

REPS:

WEIGHT USED:

CALORIES BURNED:

WATER INTAKE:

NOTES:

Just Breathe

My Workout Routine

DATE:

ACTIVITY:

TIME:

DISTANCE:

SETS:

REPS:

WEIGHT USED:

CALORIES BURNED:

WATER INTAKE:

NOTES:

Just Breathe

My Workout Routine

DATE:

ACTIVITY:

TIME:

DISTANCE:

SETS:

REPS:

WEIGHT USED:

CALORIES BURNED:

WATER INTAKE:

NOTES:

Just Breathe

My Workout Routine

DATE:

ACTIVITY:

TIME:

DISTANCE:

SETS:

REPS:

WEIGHT USED:

CALORIES BURNED:

WATER INTAKE:

NOTES:

Just Breathe

Meal Planner

WEEK OF

GROCERY LIST

- ☐
- ☐
- ☐
- ☐
- ☐
- ☐
- ☐
- ☐
- ☐
- ☐
- ☐
- ☐
- ☐
- ☐
- ☐
- ☐
- ☐
- ☐
- ☐
- ☐

MON

TUES

WED

THUR

FRI

SAT

SUN

Food Log

WEEK OF

	Breakfast	Lunch	Dinner	Snacks
Sun				
Mon				
Tues				
Wed				
Thur				
Fri				
Sat				

Thoughts . . .

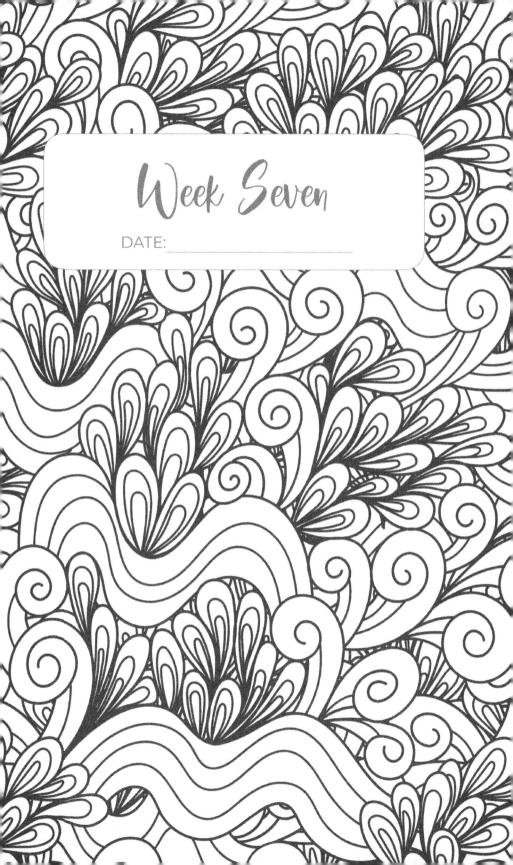

Week Seven

DATE: _____

This Week's Goals

FITNESS TO DO   **M**   **T**   **W**   **T**   **F**   **S**   **S**

Fitness Progress Tracker

DATE: _____

	MEASUREMENT:	LOSS/GAIN:
WEIGHT:		
LEFT ARM:		
RIGHT ARM:		
CHEST:		
WAIST:		
HIPS:		
LEFT THIGH:		
RIGHT THIGH:		

How's It Going?

Good things TAKE TIME

My Workout Routine

DATE:

ACTIVITY:

TIME:

DISTANCE:

SETS:

REPS:

WEIGHT USED:

CALORIES BURNED:

WATER INTAKE:

NOTES:

Just Breathe

My Workout Routine

DATE:

ACTIVITY:

TIME:

DISTANCE:

SETS:

REPS:

WEIGHT USED:

CALORIES BURNED:

WATER INTAKE:

NOTES:

Just Breathe

My Workout Routine

DATE:

ACTIVITY:

TIME:

DISTANCE:

SETS:

REPS:

WEIGHT USED:

CALORIES BURNED:

WATER INTAKE:

NOTES:

Just Breathe

My Workout Routine

DATE:

ACTIVITY:

TIME:

DISTANCE:

SETS:

REPS:

WEIGHT USED:

CALORIES BURNED:

WATER INTAKE:

NOTES:

Just Breathe

Meal Planner

WEEK OF

GROCERY LIST

- [ ]
- [ ]
- [ ]
- [ ]
- [ ]
- [ ]
- [ ]
- [ ]
- [ ]
- [ ]
- [ ]
- [ ]
- [ ]
- [ ]
- [ ]
- [ ]
- [ ]
- [ ]
- [ ]
- [ ]
- [ ]

MON

TUES

WED

THUR

FRI

SAT

SUN

Food Log

WEEK OF

	Breakfast	Lunch	Dinner	Snacks
Sun				
Mon				
Tues				
Wed				
Thur				
Fri				
Sat				

Thoughts . . .

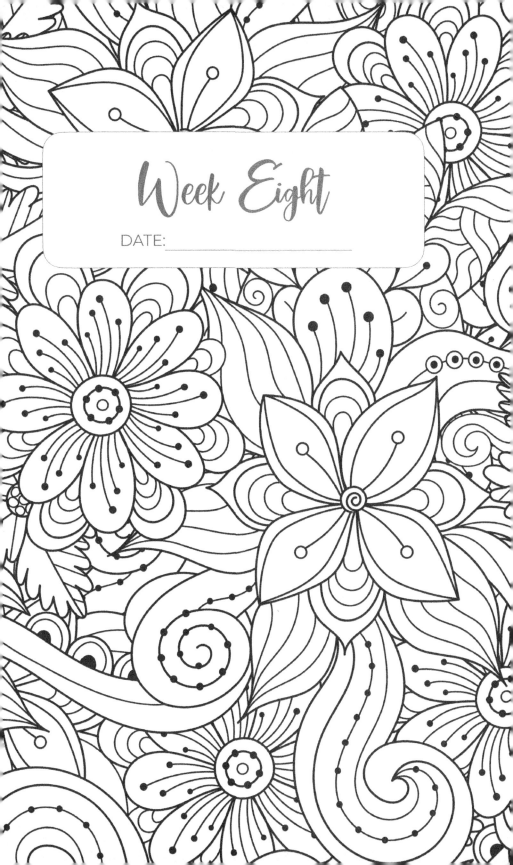

Week Eight

DATE: _____

This Week's Goals

FITNESS TO DO   **M   T   W   T   F   S   S**

Fitness Progress Tracker

DATE: ───

	MEASUREMENT:	LOSS/GAIN:
WEIGHT:		
LEFT ARM:		
RIGHT ARM:		
CHEST:		
WAIST:		
HIPS:		
LEFT THIGH:		
RIGHT THIGH:		

How's It Going?

Good things TAKE TIME

My Workout Routine

DATE:

ACTIVITY:

TIME:

DISTANCE:

SETS:

REPS:

WEIGHT USED:

CALORIES BURNED:

WATER INTAKE:

NOTES:

Just Breathe

My Workout Routine

DATE:

ACTIVITY:

TIME:

DISTANCE:

SETS:

REPS:

WEIGHT USED:

CALORIES BURNED:

WATER INTAKE:

NOTES:

Just Breathe

My Workout Routine

DATE:

ACTIVITY:

TIME:

DISTANCE:

SETS:

REPS:

WEIGHT USED:

CALORIES BURNED:

WATER INTAKE:

NOTES:

Just Breathe

My Workout Routine

DATE:

ACTIVITY:

TIME:

DISTANCE:

SETS:

REPS:

WEIGHT USED:

CALORIES BURNED:

WATER INTAKE:

NOTES:

Just Breathe

Meal Planner

GROCERY LIST

- [ ]
- [ ]
- [ ]
- [ ]
- [ ]
- [ ]
- [ ]
- [ ]
- [ ]
- [ ]
- [ ]
- [ ]
- [ ]
- [ ]
- [ ]
- [ ]
- [ ]
- [ ]
- [ ]
- [ ]

MON

TUES

WED

THUR

FRI

SAT

SUN

Food Log

WEEK OF

	Breakfast	Lunch	Dinner	Snacks
Sun				
Mon				
Tues				
Wed				
Thur				
Fri				
Sat				

Thoughts. . .

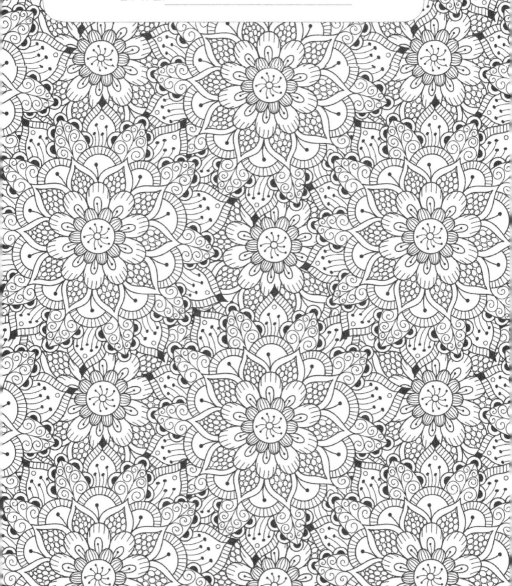

Week Nine

DATE: _____

This Week's Goals

FITNESS TO DO   M   T   W   T   F   S   S

Fitness Progress Tracker

DATE: _____

	MEASUREMENT:	LOSS/GAIN:
WEIGHT:		
LEFT ARM:		
RIGHT ARM:		
CHEST:		
WAIST:		
HIPS:		
LEFT THIGH:		
RIGHT THIGH:		

How's It Going?

Good things TAKE TIME

My Workout Routine

DATE:

ACTIVITY:

TIME:

DISTANCE:

SETS:

REPS:

WEIGHT USED:

CALORIES BURNED:

WATER INTAKE:

NOTES:

Just Breathe

My Workout Routine

DATE:

ACTIVITY:

TIME:

DISTANCE:

SETS:

REPS:

WEIGHT USED:

CALORIES BURNED:

WATER INTAKE:

NOTES:

Just Breathe

My Workout Routine

DATE:

ACTIVITY:

TIME:

DISTANCE:

SETS:

REPS:

WEIGHT USED:

CALORIES BURNED:

WATER INTAKE:

NOTES:

Just Breathe

My Workout Routine

DATE:

ACTIVITY:

TIME:

DISTANCE:

SETS:

REPS:

WEIGHT USED:

CALORIES BURNED:

WATER INTAKE:

NOTES:

Just Breathe

Meal Planner

WEEK OF

GROCERY LIST

- [ ]
- [ ]
- [ ]
- [ ]
- [ ]
- [ ]
- [ ]
- [ ]
- [ ]
- [ ]
- [ ]
- [ ]
- [ ]
- [ ]
- [ ]
- [ ]
- [ ]
- [ ]
- [ ]
- [ ]

MON

TUES

WED

THUR

FRI

SAT

SUN

Food Log

WEEK OF

	Breakfast	Lunch	Dinner	Snacks
Sun				
Mon				
Tues				
Wed				
Thur				
Fri				
Sat				

Thoughts . . .

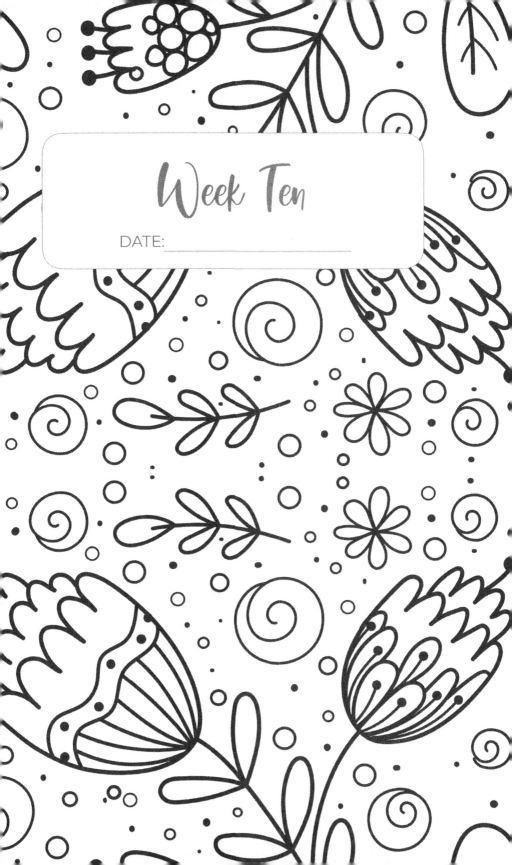

Week Ten

DATE: _____

This Week's Goals

FITNESS TO DO   M   T   W   T   F   S   S

Fitness Progress Tracker

DATE: _____

	MEASUREMENT:	LOSS/GAIN:
WEIGHT:		
LEFT ARM:		
RIGHT ARM:		
CHEST:		
WAIST:		
HIPS:		
LEFT THIGH:		
RIGHT THIGH:		

How's It Going?

Good things TAKE TIME

My Workout Routine

DATE:

ACTIVITY:

TIME:

DISTANCE:

SETS:

REPS:

WEIGHT USED:

CALORIES BURNED:

WATER INTAKE:

NOTES:

Just Breathe

My Workout Routine

DATE:

ACTIVITY:

TIME:

DISTANCE:

SETS:

REPS:

WEIGHT USED:

CALORIES BURNED:

WATER INTAKE:

NOTES:

Just Breathe

My Workout Routine

DATE:

ACTIVITY:

TIME:

DISTANCE:

SETS:

REPS:

WEIGHT USED:

CALORIES BURNED:

WATER INTAKE:

NOTES:

Just Breathe

My Workout Routine

DATE:

ACTIVITY:

TIME:

DISTANCE:

SETS:

REPS:

WEIGHT USED:

CALORIES BURNED:

WATER INTAKE:

NOTES:

Just Breathe

Meal Planner

WEEK OF

GROCERY LIST

- [ ]
- [ ]
- [ ]
- [ ]
- [ ]
- [ ]
- [ ]
- [ ]
- [ ]
- [ ]
- [ ]
- [ ]
- [ ]
- [ ]
- [ ]
- [ ]
- [ ]
- [ ]
- [ ]

MON

TUES

WED

THUR

FRI

SAT

SUN

Food Log

WEEK OF

	Breakfast	Lunch	Dinner	Snacks
Sun				
Mon				
Tues				
Wed				
Thur				
Fri				
Sat				

Thoughts. . .

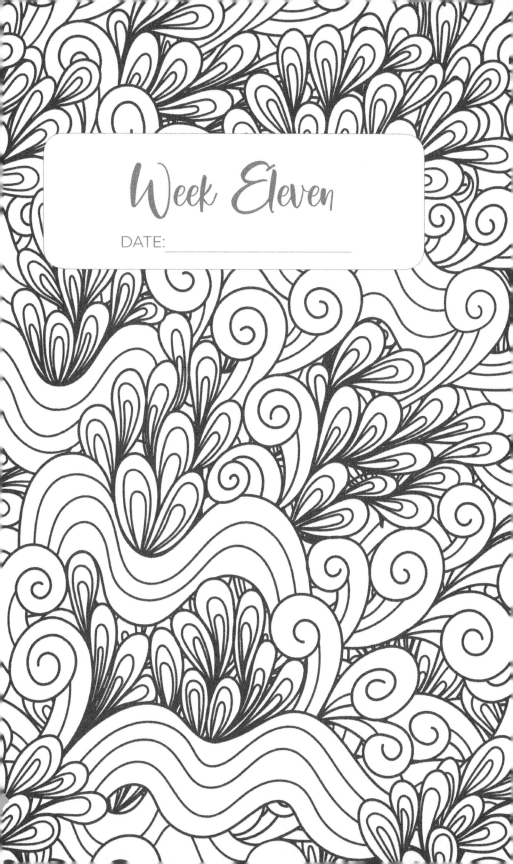

Week Eleven

DATE: _____

This Week's Goals

FITNESS TO DO   **M**   **T**   **W**   **T**   **F**   **S**   **S**

Fitness Progress Tracker

DATE: _____

	MEASUREMENT:	LOSS/GAIN:
WEIGHT:		
LEFT ARM:		
RIGHT ARM:		
CHEST:		
WAIST:		
HIPS:		
LEFT THIGH:		
RIGHT THIGH:		

How's It Going?

Good things TAKE TIME

My Workout Routine

DATE:

ACTIVITY:

TIME:

DISTANCE:

SETS:

REPS:

WEIGHT USED:

CALORIES BURNED:

WATER INTAKE:

NOTES:

Just Breathe

My Workout Routine

DATE:

ACTIVITY:

TIME:

DISTANCE:

SETS:

REPS:

WEIGHT USED:

CALORIES BURNED:

WATER INTAKE:

NOTES:

Just Breathe

My Workout Routine

DATE:

ACTIVITY:

TIME:

DISTANCE:

SETS:

REPS:

WEIGHT USED:

CALORIES BURNED:

WATER INTAKE:

NOTES:

Just Breathe

My Workout Routine

DATE:

ACTIVITY:

TIME:

DISTANCE:

SETS:

REPS:

WEIGHT USED:

CALORIES BURNED:

WATER INTAKE:

NOTES:

Just Breathe

Meal Planner

WEEK OF

GROCERY LIST

- [ ]
- [ ]
- [ ]
- [ ]
- [ ]
- [ ]
- [ ]
- [ ]
- [ ]
- [ ]
- [ ]
- [ ]
- [ ]
- [ ]
- [ ]
- [ ]
- [ ]
- [ ]
- [ ]

MON

TUES

WED

THUR

FRI

SAT

SUN

Food Log

WEEK OF

	Breakfast	Lunch	Dinner	Snacks
Sun				
Mon				
Tues				
Wed				
Thur				
Fri				
Sat				

Thoughts. . .

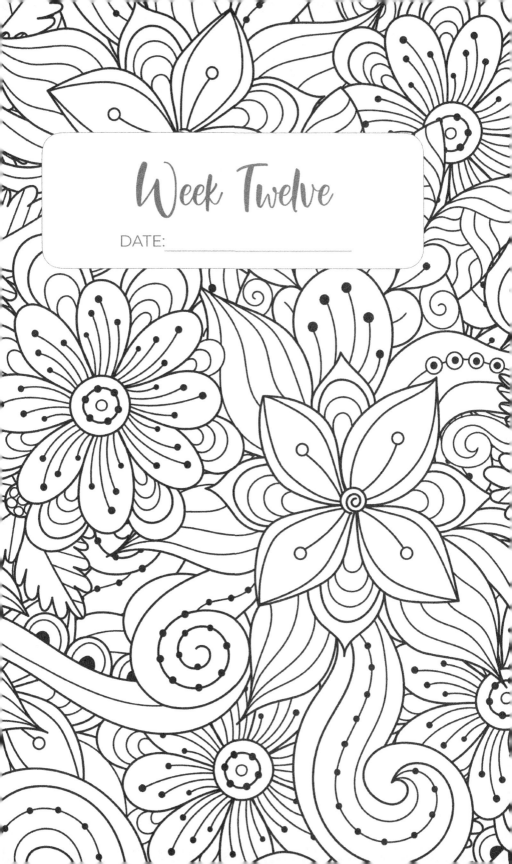

Week Twelve

DATE:_____

This Week's Goals

FITNESS TO DO   **M   T   W   T   F   S   S**

Fitness Progress Tracker

DATE: _____

	MEASUREMENT:	LOSS/GAIN:
WEIGHT:		
LEFT ARM:		
RIGHT ARM:		
CHEST:		
WAIST:		
HIPS:		
LEFT THIGH:		
RIGHT THIGH:		

How's It Going?

Good things TAKE TIME

My Workout Routine

DATE:

ACTIVITY:

TIME:

DISTANCE:

SETS:

REPS:

WEIGHT USED:

CALORIES BURNED:

WATER INTAKE:

NOTES:

Just Breathe

My Workout Routine

DATE:

ACTIVITY:

TIME:

DISTANCE:

SETS:

REPS:

WEIGHT USED:

CALORIES BURNED:

WATER INTAKE:

NOTES:

Just Breathe

My Workout Routine

DATE:

ACTIVITY:

TIME:

DISTANCE:

SETS:

REPS:

WEIGHT USED:

CALORIES BURNED:

WATER INTAKE:

NOTES:

Just Breathe

My Workout Routine

DATE:

ACTIVITY:

TIME:

DISTANCE:

SETS:

REPS:

WEIGHT USED:

CALORIES BURNED:

WATER INTAKE:

NOTES:

Just Breathe

Meal Planner

GROCERY LIST

- [ ]
- [ ]
- [ ]
- [ ]
- [ ]
- [ ]
- [ ]
- [ ]
- [ ]
- [ ]
- [ ]
- [ ]
- [ ]
- [ ]
- [ ]
- [ ]
- [ ]
- [ ]
- [ ]

MON

TUES

WED

THUR

FRI

SAT

SUN

Food Log

WEEK OF

	Breakfast	Lunch	Dinner	Snacks
Sun				
Mon				
Tues				
Wed				
Thu				
Fri				
Sat				

Thoughts. . .

12 - Week Total Weight Log

CURRENT:

PREVIOUS:

CHANGE:

NOTES

Good things TAKE TIME

Congratulations!

You Did It!

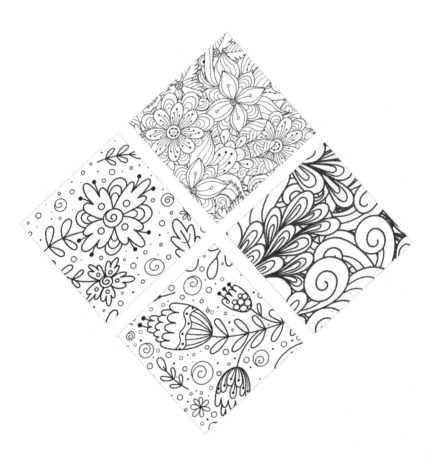

Now It's Time To Play. . .

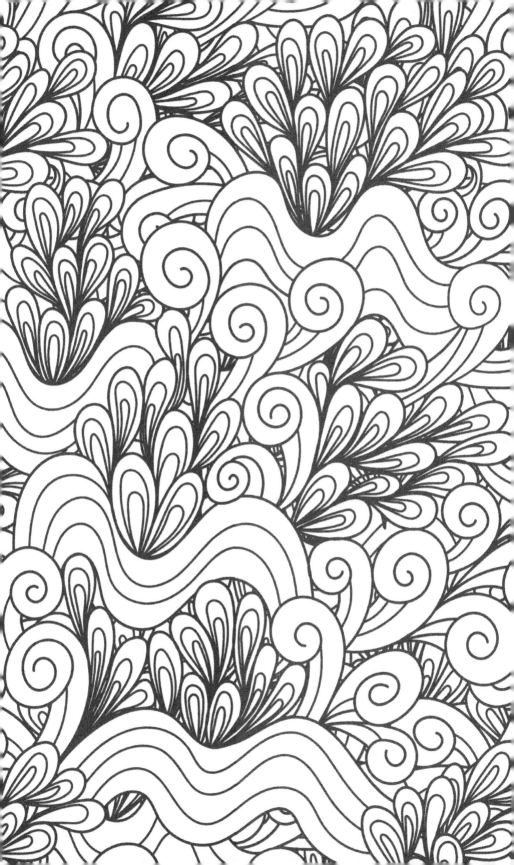

Made in the USA
Monee, IL
22 February 2022